Medical Disclaimer

Acknowledgements

I would like to thank all the people who have made this book possible:

My gratitude to Michio Kushi, Herman Aihara, and Steven Acuff for teaching the five elements and how they relate to diet and health.

Thanks to Shou-yu Liang and Wen-Ching Wu for their teaching on medical Qigong.

My gratitude to Connie Kroskin for designing what was a 5-hour seminar into this beautiful book. Thanks for the artwork she contributed as well.

I am grateful for the careful editing by Elizabeth Binder while also helping to run a busy office.

Thanks to Caroline Danielson for her wonderful work on the final editing.

My wife, Paivi, for producing the beautiful pastel artwork for each element.

My thanks to all my patients and their organs for teaching me so much about how the body can heal. Gratitude to God and to all the invisible beings who assist me in my work.

Warren King

Foreward

Imagine that you had 10 servants that had as their life mission to keep you happy and healthy. They would work for you, keep you feeling positive, throw out the garbage, and perform hundreds of other tasks. You do have these servants. They are the 10 main organs of your body.

In this book you will learn the language these organs use to communicate with you. Now your symptoms will make sense and you will understand what your organs have been trying to tell you.

Ancient Chinese healers discovered the forces of the universe and how the 5 basic energies or "elements" relate to our organs and our health. In this full-color book you will find many tools, such as facial diagnosis, acupressure, cooking, herbology, and qigong, that will help you on the road to regaining or maintaining your health. You will discover the amazing connection between each organ and specific emotions.

Warren King has been a licensed acupuncturist for over 23 years and has treated over 8000 patients. He has developed his intuition to be able to communicate with the intelligence of the body and the energy of the organs. Now he combines the ancient healing wisdom of the East with the modern understanding of how our organs work and puts it all together in this book, a feast for the eyes and the mind.

Included is a bonus chapter, "America the Toxic," which describes how modern toxins are affecting our health in ways that the ancient healers could never have anticipated.

Table of Contents

Bonus...

About the Elements

fire

earth

metal

wood

water

The Ancient Chinese

- They carefully observed nature.
- They noted the flow of energy in the universe.
- They applied this to an energy-based medicine.
- This medicine has practical use in healing the body and mind.

The Tai Chi or Yin / Yang

- Everything in existence has a polarity.
- There are dual energies within the circle of the one wholeness, the Tao.
- We call them yin and yang.

Everything Has Polarity

- Expansive and contractive
- Hot and cold
- Light and dark
- Male and female
- Outside and inside
- Positive and negative

Yin Within Yang, Yang Within Yin

✸ Notice the dots within the two halves.

✸ Nothing is absolute; within yin there is yang,
and yang within yin.

✸ When something goes to the extreme it turns into its
opposite.

   When you inhale all the way, you must exhale.
   When you exhale all the way, you must inhale.

**There is a flow of energy in the universe, and if you go with
the current it can be fun.** You can try the sidestroke or the
backstroke. But if you go against the flow, it's hard work. You
get illness and have no energy for psychological and spiritual
development.

Try to understand life as energy. In physics, matter is not
thought of as solid but as condensed energy. That energy has 2
types: expansive and contractive. Your heart and lungs and cells
are continuously expanding and contracting.

Stress is yang and tightening, so some people reach for alcohol,
which is yin and expansive. See if you can find better ways
to achieve the balance your body is seeking. **We have to
experiment on ourselves to find out how to balance these
energies.**

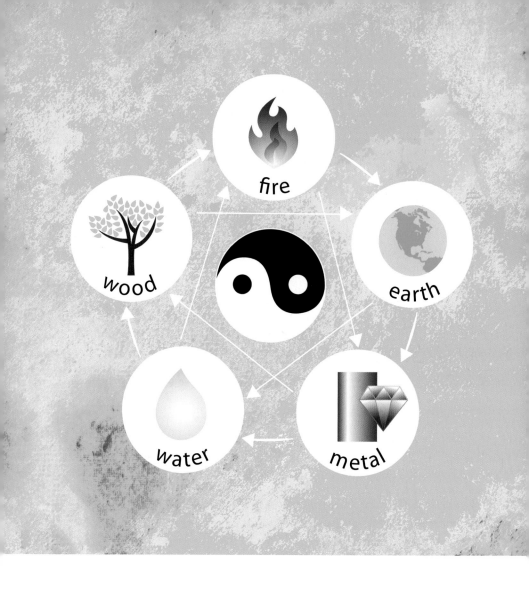

The 5 Elements

⊛ Yin and yang can be broken into 5 parts.

⊛ They are often called the elements.

⊛ They can be called the 5 phases of energy.

⊛ The movement of energy from expansion to contraction, and from contraction to expansion.

Cycling of the 5 Elements

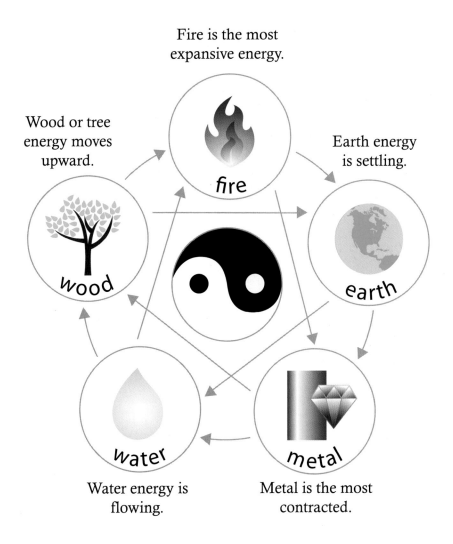

Fire is the most expansive energy.

Wood or tree energy moves upward.

Earth energy is settling.

fire

wood

earth

water

metal

Water energy is flowing.

Metal is the most contracted.

5 Elements and Health

- The Chinese applied the 5 elements to the body.

- This became the basis of Oriental medicine.

- There is a yin/yang organ pair for each element.

- One organ is usually solid, and the paired organ is hollow.

Acupuncture Meridians

❋ Each organ is associated with an energy flow along the surface of the skin.

❋ When the energy is flowing smoothly in the meridians and organs, there is health.

❋ When the energy is stagnated, excessive, or deficient, there is illness.

7

Modifying Energy Flow

The energy flow can be manipulated by various means:

- Acupuncture needles

- Acupressure

- Heat (moxibustion)

- Suction with cupping

- Modern methods
such as electricity,
crystals or gems,
infrared heat,
magnetism
or lasers

The Earth Element
Spleen, Pancreas, and Stomach

Earth

The acrid scent of compost pile
The diaper of a newborn child

Earth, just turned, in garden bed
The roses of the newly wed

The freshest air, when storm has passed
The fragrance of the fresh cut grass

I bring the fire of life to form
Your soul with flesh I do adorn

Between the seasons I give you rest
Truly I am the cosmic breast

I would not have you burn your lips
You must have reality in tiny sips

A handful of dirt that teems with life
If you like, I am spirit's wife

In volcanic ash new life shall creep
Pollen sprouting to pistil's deep

The softness of each petal rare
Floral fragrance distilled with care

My joy to serve, as farmer's toil
All you need springs from my soil.

—Warren King

Energy of Earth

Think of it as energy settling down

When the fire has passed its peak and ashes form, creating earth.

Energy is moving downward, coalescing, like the formation of compost

Like water coming down as rain.

Earth in the Daily Cycle

✳ Because earth energy is downward, it has to do with afternoon, so earth rules the energy of afternoon.

✳ Do you feel your energy drop in the afternoon? That is due to a blood sugar drop, which is related to the pancreas or spleen in Eastern medicine.

Earth in the Yearly Cycle

Indian summer is like the afternoon of the year

Not quite summer, but not quite fall

Earth is also seen as the cycle of transition between every season

12

Earth Element Organs

Earth corresponds to the spleen and pancreas.

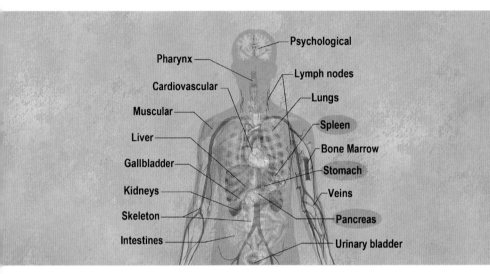

Psychological

Pharynx

Lymph nodes

Cardiovascular

Lungs

Muscular

Spleen

Liver

Bone Marrow

Gallbladder

Stomach

Kidneys

Veins

Skeleton

Pancreas

Intestines

Urinary bladder

The spleen acts as a filter against foreign organisms that infect the bloodstream. It also filters out old red blood cells from the bloodstream and decomposes them.

The spleen also acts as a blood reservoir. It manufactures red blood cells at the end of fetal development.

The pancreas is yellowish, 7 inches long, and is behind the stomach. It releases 3 digestive enzymes into the small intestine to break down carbohydrates, proteins, and fats.

The islets of Langerhans, a region within the pancreas, secretes two hormones, insulin and glucagon. Insulin lowers the blood sugar level and increases the amount of glycogen (stored carbohydrate) in the liver; glucagon has the opposite action.

When the cells stop producing insulin, you have diabetes. When cells stop responding to insulin, you have insulin resistance.

Paired Organ of Earth

The hollow organ that is paired with the spleen is the stomach.

Liver — Stomach
Duodenum — Gall Bladder
Pancreas — Spleen
Ascending Colon — Transverse Colon
Small Intestine — Large Intestine
Appendix — Rectum
— Anus

The stomach is about 12 inches long and 6 inches wide at its widest point. Its capacity is about 1 quart in an adult.

The surface of the mucosa is honeycombed with over 35,000 gastric glands that secrete hydrochloric acid. The stomach churns the food, but proper chewing, which mixes the food with saliva, begins digestion of starches and is needed to make the particles small enough for proper digestion.

Blood sugar problems are not all from sugar, but are also from fat. High fat content in blood dulls insulin's effectiveness. Overweight people are more likely to become diabetic. Most people of average weight are less likely to need insulin.

Fats tighten the pancreas so that it becomes less effective. French fries, greasy foods, and heavy animal fats can lead to blood sugar problems. Ice-cold foods and drinks shock the stomach and pancreas. Americans consume ice-cold water and ice cream all year round, even in winter.

Body Part Association

Each organ is associated with, or considered to rule, a certain body part and sense organ. **The spleen rules the muscles.**

The spleen is connected to the pancreas, and one symptom of diabetes is wasting of the muscles.

Image: Patrick J. Lynch; medical illustrator; C. Carl Jaffe, MD, cardiologist

Sense Organ Association

The spleen corresponds to the mouth and lips.

Cold sores on the lips can be associated with a spleen imbalance.

The Taste of Earth

The flavor associated with the spleen,
pancreas, and stomach is sweet.

No flavor causes more problems than sweet. Is like a drug that people want to get off of, can go months without, then go to a family gathering, try some, and suddenly need it daily.

Complex carbohydrates give strength, but simple sugars should be kept to a minimum. They rob the body of B vitamins, disturb mineral balance, rot teeth and make the body tissues acid.

Blood sugar constantly fluctuates. When it's down, we crave sweet. Eating a candy bar is like throwing gasoline on a fire; you get a quick kick but have nothing left afterwards.

When your blood sugar is low, you can try a more complex sweetener like rice syrup or barley malt. If you need a quick sugar, you can try a tropical fruit.

The long-term solution is to add sweet vegetables to your diet: carrots, parsnips, rutabagas, squash, yams, sweet potatoes, and other good, complex sugars.

Fiber slows absorption, so if you need sugar faster you can have vegetable juice or fruit juice. Also if you have low blood sugar like hypoglycemia, whole grains are good. If you want to raise it faster have some bread.

A sweet vegetable drink is a great home remedy to help with blood sugar imbalances. Drinking a broth made from sweet vegetables also alkalizes the body, balancing an excess acid state.

When you have a heavy meal you'll want something yin, sweet, and light after to balance it, so have some cooked berries or applesauce. If you have something more yang with heavy stuff like baked flour and oils, you'll still feel heavy and continue craving sweets.

The purpose of dessert is to be light, not heavy. Sluggish, overweight individuals or those with dampness, such as excess mucus should take sweets very sparingly, and even whole food carbohydrates moderately. Chewing carbohydrates well makes them less mucus forming.

Spleen/Pancreas and Sweets

When sugar enters the system, the pancreas secretes insulin to open the cells to the sugar.

Artificial sweeteners can cause diabetes by throwing off the balance of bacteria in the intestines.

Complex carbohydrates break down more slowly in the system, creating less of a blood sugar spike, and therefore, less of an emotional roller coaster.

Nourishing Earth Foods

Grains

Millet

Squashes

Onions

Sweet fruits

Blueberries

Figs

Dates

Honey

Rice syrup

Barley malt

Cooking Styles

Roasting

Stewing

Beating

Mashing

Purees

Jams & Jellies

Desserts

Herbs for Stomach

Chamomile

Ginger

Peppermint

Alfalfa

Stevia

Dandelion Root

The Spleen and Emotions

- Thought, mental function and concentration have to do with the spleen.

- Empathy, understanding, and compassion are signs of a balanced earth element.

- An imbalanced earth element can produce over-thinking and worry.

If the spleen is out of balance you feel anxious, worried, and too sympathetic or sensitive.

When in balance you feel calm, soothed, more discriminating and self-determined. You feel like singing.

When you have a healthy stomach, it results in mental and emotional stability, while imbalance leads to worry, skepticism, and anxiety.

The Spirit of the Spleen

❂ The Spirit that incarnates in the spleen is called the Yi.

❂ The Yi has to do with intention, purpose, clarity of thought, altruism, and integrity.

❂ Chronic worrying and rumination are signs of an imbalanced Yi.

The Yi represents the power of the earth in us. It is the spirit that gives us the capacity for sustained intention, purpose, clarity of thought, altruism, and integrity. It is related to the emotions of sympathy and the organ of the spleen.

It supports our capacity for thought, intention, reflection, and the act of applying ourselves to our heart's purpose.

It gives us the ability to concentrate, study, and memorize data for one's work, and endows us with the capacity for clear thought. **In other words, it allows us to apply our spirit to the world of form.**

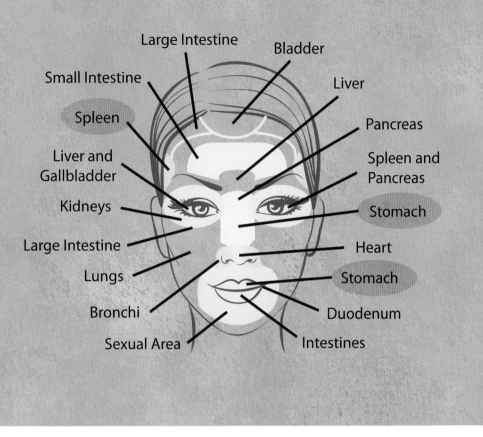

Large Intestine
Bladder
Small Intestine
Liver
Spleen
Pancreas
Liver and Gallbladder
Spleen and Pancreas
Kidneys
Stomach
Large Intestine
Heart
Lungs
Stomach
Bronchi
Duodenum
Sexual Area
Intestines

Facial Diagnosis

🞉 **The face never lies.**

🞉 The bridge of the nose is the stomach.

🞉 The eyelids reflect the state of the spleen.

The stomach is reflected in the upper lip and bridge of the nose. A swollen upper lip is caused by refined carbohydrates, fruit, alcohol, or white flour.

A contracted stomach can be seen in a tight upper lip and can be from meat, eggs, salt, dry baked food, or fasting. Blood vessels expanded on the eyelids or styes can indicate a spleen imbalance.

SP 20
SP 19
SP 18
SP 17
SP 21
SP 16
SP 15
SP 14
SP 13
SP 12
SP 11
SP 10
SP 9
SP 8
SP 7
SP 6
SP 5
SP 4
SP 3
SP 2
SP 1

The Spleen Meridian

- From outside of big toe to chest.

- 21 acupuncture points.

- The spleen governs the transportation and transformation of nutrients, helping food become qi, or life force energy, and blood.

- It has to do with digestion, and a dysfunction leads to bloating, diarrhea, and lack of appetite.

Some problems related to the spleen meridian can be big toe issues, inner knee pain, swelling of the inner leg, diaphragm issues, and esophagus or tongue symptoms.

Internal pathway blockages can create diaphragm and lung conditions, tightness in the chest, feeling of something in the throat (plum pit), and eye pain.

25

ST 8
ST 7
ST 6
ST 5
ST 9
ST 10
ST 11
ST 12
ST 13
ST 14
ST 15
ST 16
ST 17
ST 18
ST 19
ST 20
ST 21
ST 22
ST 23
ST 24
ST 25
ST 26
ST 27
ST 28
ST 29
ST 30
ST 31
ST 32
ST 33
ST 34
ST 35
ST 36
ST 37
ST 38
ST 40
ST 39
ST 41
ST 42
ST 43
ST 44
ST 45

Stomach Meridian

❋ From the eye to the 2nd toe.

❋ 45 acupuncture points.

❋ The stomach initiates the metabolism of food and drink.

2nd and 3rd toe are the end of the stomach meridian. If they are longer than the big toe and webbed, this indicates excess fruit, sugar, medications, or refined foods during pregnancy, giving an expanded, or yin, stomach.

If these 2 toes are much shorter than the big toe or bend toward the big toe, your mother may have eaten too much salt or animal food during pregnancy.

Vigorous massage of these 2 toes helps nausea or stomach upset.

Meridian imbalances can create cheek marks, throat issues, breast issues, digestive and ovarian issues, pain or skin issues on area of the legs where the meridian runs, knee pain, and acid reflux or frequent hunger.

26

Acu Point for Spleen

Spleen 6-Sanyinjiao-three yin junction (liver, kidney, and spleen channels meet at this point).

Location: Put 4 fingers together and measure this length above the inner ankle bone, point is located just behind the bone (tibia).

Benefits: Poor digestion, insomnia, anemia, water retention, menstrual or female organ problems, calms the spirit.

For acupressure, use your middle or index finger at a 90 degree angle to the points. Apply firm and steady pressure. This may be tender but shouldn't be painful. Hold the point for about 3 minutes. You can also visualize light coming out of your finger and illuminating the meridian and the associated organ.

Stomach Acu Point

Stomach 36-Zusanli-leg three miles

Location: 4 finger lengths below kneecap on the outside of the tibia, 1 finger length from the bone.

Benefits: Strengthens energy of the whole body, helps digestion, circulation, anxiety, headaches and leg pain.

Time of Day Earth Meridians Peak

12

11

10

Energy peaks in the spleen channel at 9-11 AM.

9

Energy peaks in the stomach channel at 7-9 AM.

8

7

Energy travels in the acupuncture organs and meridians throughout the day in a 24-hour period.

It is interesting that we should be eating and digesting breakfast in the peak times for the stomach and spleen. Research is really showing how eating a good breakfast is a key for weight and blood sugar and for learning, all earth element issues.

6

Healing Sound for the Spleen

Qigong has a healing sound for the major organs, *Hu* is the sound for the spleen (whooo).

STEP 1: Stand naturally upright. Inhale and bring your hands next to your breast area with your palms facing up and fingers pointing at each other. During inhalation, imagine leading the energy from your big toe on your left foot up the inside of your left leg and up to your spleen.

STEP 2: Exhale and rotate your right palm out and up. Rotate your left palm in and down, then extend your right hand up and your left hand down. When exhaling, imagine leading impurities from your spleen out, passing a point at your left armpit, then down to a point just below the left rib cage. When exhaling, make the *Hu* sound. While drawing your stomach and the center of the perineum in and up, squeeze out the impurities from your spleen.

STEP 3: Inhale and bring both hands down facing each other like in Step 1. Next, rotate your left palm out and up then rotate your right palm in and down. Next, extend your left palm up and your right palm down. Exhale as you did on the other side. During inhalation, imagine leading the energy from your left big toe up the inside of your left leg and up to your spleen. Repeat a total of 6 inhalations and exhalations.

The Metal Element
Lung and Large Intestine

Metal

Those on earth call me real
No phantasm or cloud with me you'll feel

Hit your thumb with a hammer, bang!
I am the essence who is most Yang

Those of the east named me metal
Perhaps the new age shall call me crystal

Strength and tension, pressure and strain
The bone of form, the skull for your brain

God's kindgom extended to the realms most dense
Valiant souls then journeyed hence

The fist of the victor, the diamond, the will
The spine of a cactus, an avalanche spill

To air I am thunder to water I'm hail
My iron stokes fires, to wood I'm the nail

To earth I'm the shovel, I'm the essence of men
The bullet, the sword blade, the tip of the pen

The teeth of the lion, the nails of a hare
Feel my action if indeed you dare!

—Warren King

Energy of Metal

Don't think of it as a piece of metal

Think of it more like the most contracted energy

It could be metal or a stone or a crystal

...or water freezing into ice

Metal in the Daily Cycle

▼ Since metal is downward energy, it has to do with the sunset.

▼ So metal rules the energy of evening.

▼ Think of how you start going within at dusk.

▼ Do you feel like crashing after work?

Metal in the Yearly Cycle

▼ Fall is like the sunset of the year.

▼ Everything is moving inward and downward.

▼ If you feel worse in the fall with allergies,
for example, you could be experiencing
a metal imbalance.

Metal Element Organs

Metal corresponds to the lungs

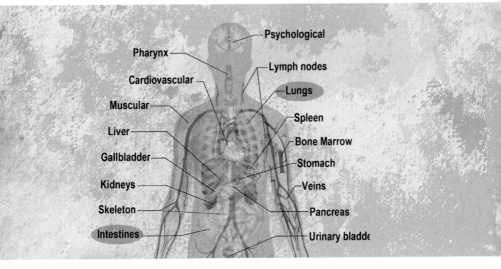

▼ At rest, a person breathes about 14 to 16 times per minute. During exercise it could increase to over 60 times per minute.

▼ New babies at rest breathe between 40 and 50 times per minute. By age 5 it decreases to around 25 times per minute.

▼ The total surface area of the alveoli (tiny air sacs in the lungs) is the size of a tennis court.

▼ The lungs are the only organ in the body that can float on water.

Paired Organ of Metal

The hollow organ paired with the lungs is the large intestine

▼ The large intestine is about 5 feet long. The appendix hangs off the large intestine, and scientists are only beginning to understand that it is a reservoir for the beneficial flora in the large intestine.

▼ We have as many bacteria in our large intestine as cells in our bodies, about 75 trillion, and over 400 species of micro-organisms.

▼ Water and some vitamins and minerals are reabsorbed from the waste that moves on to become stool.

▼ It can take food 3 days to move through the 15 feet of the gastrointestinal tract. In other cultures it can take 4-6 hours due to a better diet, more exercise and less stress.

- 70% of the cells that make up the body's immune system are found in the wall of the gut.
- When parasites or yeast (candida) overgrow in the intestines you can get systemic health problems.
- Intestinal problems are often the forerunner of other health problems and chronic constipation is a pre-warning sign for cancer, especially for breasts, which are over the lungs and connected energetically with the large intestine.

Large intestine health issues:
- Crohn's disease
- Colitis
- Irritable bowel
- Gas
- Bloating
- Constipation
- Diarrhea
- Hemorrhoids
- Colon cancer
- Toxic intestines can create many skin conditions.
- Sinus problems are often associated with the intestines as well. Psoriasis and asthma often go together; when one is suppressed it may lead to the other.

Our intestines are overfed, overworked and under exercised.

Body Part Association

Each organ is associated with, or considered to rule, a certain body part and sense organ. **Lungs rule the skin.**

Lungs have to do with what is called the wei chi or defensive energy of the body that surrounds the skin. Sweating is thought to be related to the lungs, so it is no surprise that those who take saunas in the winter have fewer colds. Many Chinese herb formulas for infections have diaphoretic herbs, or herbs that promote sweating. Thus the invading wind and cold are pushed outward so the infection doesn't go deeper.

Image: Todtanis

Sense Organ Association

The lungs correspond to the nose.

The nose and sinuses are all considered part of the lung energy system.

The Taste of Metal

The flavor associated with the lung
and large intestine is pungent.

Pungent
flavors, like
ginger, are
very good
for digestion.
This flavor
dispels
mucus from
the lung
and large
intestine.

Nourishing Metal Foods

Examples of nourishing metal foods...

Onions	Leeks
Garlic	Chinese cabbage
Ginger	Bok choy
Daikon radish	Celery
Peppers	Cucumber
Red radishes	Spicy peppers
Chives	Rice

▼ Dairy can produce mucus, as can flour products like breads, cookies, cakes and muffins. If you eat more than a moderate portion or don't chew well, your body will produce mucus and your food will not be properly digested.

Pungent foods clear mucus from the lungs, improve digestion, and expel gas from the intestines. They moisten the kidneys, affecting the fluids of the whole body. Thus they increase saliva and sweat.

▼ Whole grain bread can be healthy, but if you have mucus in the sinuses or lungs it's best to cut it out of your diet

If you eat too many baked flour products, which are yang, they will slow digestion and produce mucus. To counterbalance this effect, add these vegetables, which are good-quality yin and balance out dairy as well.

▼ Metal foods stimulate blood circulation and tonify the heart. They clear obstructions and improve sluggish liver function.

Those who are dull, sluggish, lethargic, or too heavy, as well as those with dampness or mucus in the lungs and large intestine are benefited by pungent foods.

The vegetables listed above can help if you feel mentally unclear or unfocused.

Photograph: Hedwig Storch

Metal Cooking Styles

Preparation: Kinpira, a Japanese cooking style in which matchstick-cut veggies are braised in oil, then water is added, and pressure-cooked.

Remember, metal is the most yang element. Dense root vegetables cut into little matchsticks is a very yang cutting style.

Pressure cooking in metal cookware and adding lots of inward pressure imparts a strong yang force. The opposite, and most yin type of cooking, is microwaving in which food is heated by exploding water molecules.

Pressure cooking grains such as rice, which is the grain for metal, and vegetables and beans makes them very soft and digestible, which soothes the mucous membranes of the lungs, sinuses, and large intestine.

Try cooking kinpira with carrots and burdock root, which is the most yang root there is. Burdock root can grow 3 feet long and can break rocks.

Lung / Large Intestine and Health

Often the lungs and sinuses reflect the condition of the large intestine.

Make sure that parasites, yeast, fungus, and bad bacteria are eliminated from the large intestine.

Fermented foods can help replenish the beneficial flora in the large intestine.

Examples are sauerkraut, kimchi, kombucha, yogurt, kefir, miso, and sourdough bread.

Herbs for Lungs

✓ Astragalus
✓ Fennel
✓ Goldenseal
✓ Licorice
✓ Thyme

The Lungs/Large Intestine and Emotions

▼ The lungs are the seat of our feelings and sentiments, and allow us to feel sadness and grief.

▼ When the lungs are weak, one tends toward self-pity, quietude, inwardness, depression, lack of will and vitality, or antisocial behavior.

▼ When the lungs are hyperactive, one is more outwardly expressive of sadness and grief with crying, sobbing, verbal pessimism or lashing out at others.

▼ Positive metal emotion includes discerning what is healthy and essential, and discerning what to take in and what to let go of.

It's interesting that lungs are the only organ we can directly control, and **crying and laughing are just strange ways of breathing.**

In the East, spirituality, meditation, and consciousness-raising involves control of the breath. So when lungs are an issue, you can feel lethargic and have difficulty thinking clearly. **When they are balanced, you feel more compassionate, energized, organized, and decisive.**

The Spirit of the Lungs

The Spirit that incarnates in the lungs is called the Po.

The Po is our embodied knowing, our animal wit, our street smarts.

It is closely related to the autonomic nervous system, the sensory receptors, especially the skin.

The Po is the part of us that can sniff out what's right or wrong, good or bad, safe or unsafe.

Deep below the level of our conscious ability to articulate in words what we think about a person, place, or situation, the Po spirit already knows, and whether or not we realize it, our body has begun to respond by contracting or expanding, hardening or softening.

Spending time with animals can help you tune into your Po, the animal soul within us.

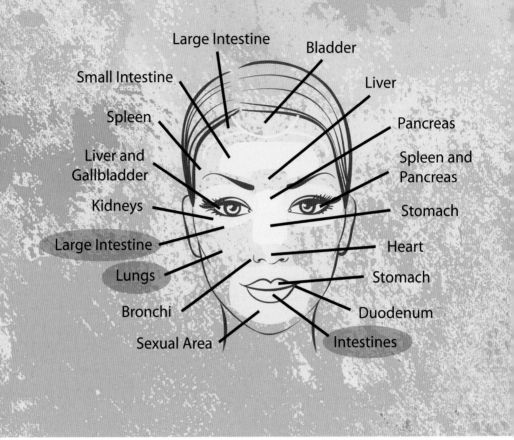

Large Intestine

Bladder

Small Intestine

Liver

Spleen

Pancreas

Liver and
Gallbladder

Spleen and
Pancreas

Kidneys

Stomach

Large Intestine

Heart

Lungs

Stomach

Bronchi

Duodenum

Sexual Area

Intestines

Facial Diagnosis

▼ **The face never lies.**

▼ The cheeks tell us about the condition of the lungs.

▼ The large intestine is reflected in the state of the lower lip.

Facial Diagnosis

Lungs are represented in the lower cheeks
at the level of the mouth.

Pimples: saturated animal fat, milk products, and sugar

White cheeks: milk products

Red: excess fruits, juices, stimulants, spices, sugar

Brown blotches: acid, mostly sugar, can be precancerous

Green: Tendency towards cancer

Moles: animal protein

Beauty marks: past fever in the lungs

Swollen lower lip: refined carbohydrates, fruit, alcohol
or white flour.

Tight lower lip: contracted large intestine from meat,
eggs, salt, dry baked food, or fasting

The condition of the intestine can also be seen in the forehead,
with the small intestine in the middle and the large
intestine around the outside.

LU 2
LU 1

LU 3
LU 4

LU 5

LU 6

LU 7
LU 8
LU 9

LU 10

LU 11

The Lung Meridian

▼ From below the clavicle or collarbone, down inside of the arm to outside corner of the thumb.

▼ 11 acupuncture points.

▼ The lung governs respiration and the extraction of Qi from the air and plays a role in fluid metabolism.

Combines Qi of air with Qi of food and spreads it throughout body via meridians and blood.

Also distributes defensive or wei chi under the skin for protection against pathogens (our immunity), so sweating is an elimination and defense ruled by the lungs.

Lung symptoms are:

shortness of breath

chest tightness

asthma

coughing

pain or skin issues along the meridian

pain in the thumbs or problems with the thumbnail

LI 20
LI 19
LI 18
LI 17
LI 16
LI 15
LI 14
LI 13
LI 12
LI 11
LI 10
LI 9
LI 8
LI 7
LI 6
LI 5
LI 4
LI 3
LI 2
LI 1

The Large Intestine Meridian

▼ From the index finger to the nose.

▼ 21 acupuncture points.

▼ The large intestine has to do with the absorption of water from food and excretion of feces.

Problems along the meridian can affect nose, lips and throat, shoulder, elbow, and wrist.

I treated a child who picked at his index finger nail until he made a hole right through it. It turned out that he had a parasite in his large intestine.

Now that you know that the large intestine rules the index finger, you can understand why nobody likes it pointed at them while being reprimanded!

Lung Acu Point
Lung 1-Zhongfu-Central Treasury

Location: Under the shoulder end of the collarbone, one hand width above the armpit, and one finger length inward.

Benefits: All lung problems, cough, asthma, congestion and phlegm. Skin problems, emotional tension, sore throat, shoulder and upper back pain.

For acupressure, use your mid or index finger at a 90 degree angle to the points. Apply firm and steady pressure, it may be tender but shouldn't be painful. Hold the point for about 3 minutes. You can also visualize light coming out of your finger and illuminating the meridian and the associated organ.

Large Intestine Acu Point

Large Intestine 4-Hegu-Joining of the Valleys

Location: In the web between the thumb and index finger on the back of the hand. At the highest point of the mound when these two digits are brought together.

Benefits: Allergies, sinus problems, headaches, itching, colds, and upper body.

Time of Day Metal Meridians Peak

Energy travels in the acupuncture organs and meridians throughout the day in a 24-hour period.

Energy peaks in the lung channel at 3 AM to 5 AM.

Energy peaks in the large intestine channel at 5AM to 7 AM.

If you can't sleep at these hours, it could indicate a blockage of the organ and meridian.

12 1 2 4 5 6 7 1

Healing Sound for Lungs

Qigong has a healing sound for the major organs. *Si* is the sound for nourishing the lungs (seeeee).

STEP 1: Stand or sit with your feet shoulder width apart, arms to your sides. Pay attention to your exhalation 3 times to remove the impurities from your lungs. Take a deep breath and imagine leading the energy (Qi) from the universe into your body, down to your 2nd toe of your right foot.

STEP 2: Hold your breath. Raise your hands up in front of your body with your hands facing up and fingers pointing toward each other. When they reach the breast area, rotate your palms until they are facing out. As you raise your hands, imagine leading the energy from the 2nd toe up the inside of your right leg and right front of your body into the lungs.

STEP 3: Exhale and begin making the *Si* (seeee) sound. At the same time, push your arms to the sides as your hold up the center of the perineum and bring your abdomen in. As you make the *Si* sound, lead the impurities out of your lungs through your mouth and down the inside of your right arm going out of your thumbnail.

Repeat Steps 1 to 3, six times.

The Wood Element
Liver and Gallbladder

Wood

The essence of a sprouting grain
Call me wood or tree, it's just a name

An upward rising energy
You may call me ascending chi

Grass, flowers or the mighty oak
I'm the power behind all growth

Though I'm the essence of all humor
When blocked I can even grow a tumor

Present at spring, I give rebirth
Behind all laughter, I am mirth

Upward and onward, my motto and song
I see what's right and not what's wrong

I wake each bird and every child
I'm in the wind that runneth wild

The mist that rises in the morn
Each new day is the sun reborn

For all those yearning to be free
Look within and look to me.

—Warren King

Energy of Wood

Don't think of wood energy as a piece of wood

Think of it more as a living tree.

Energy is moving upward, like sap moves up a tree.

Or water evaporating into clouds.

If you have a hard time waking up in the morning, it is likely that the gentle upward energy of wood is not free flowing.

Wood in the Daily Cycle

- Since wood is upward energy,
  it has to do with the sunrise.

- Wood rules the energy of the morning.

- Think of birds singing in the morning.

- Is it hard to wake up?

Wood in the Yearly Cycle

- Spring is like the sunrise of the year.

- Everything is moving upward.

- If you feel worse in the spring, such as having allergies, you could have a wood imbalance.

The liver is the largest and most complex organ of the body.

- The liver affects nearly every physiological process of the body and performs over 500 different chemical functions.

- 1/3 of all blood in the body passes through the liver every minute, about 1.5 quarts. It detoxifies the blood by filtering out toxins that assault your body on a regular basis.

- It also helps with hormonal balance, fat regulation, and digestion.

- Carbohydrates, fats, and proteins can all be changed into one another by the liver. Excess food that is not used can be turned into fat or mucus.

- If 80% of the liver is destroyed by sickness or surgery, it can grow back quickly, all the while carrying on its normal functions.

- The liver stores certain vitamins, minerals, and sugars and produces quick energy when it is needed.

- It controls the production and excretion of cholesterol, and produces immune factors than help the body fight off infection.

You should be able to get your fingers underneath your right rib cage. If it's like cement you may have compacted fat in the liver.

Wood Element Organs

Wood corresponds to the liver.

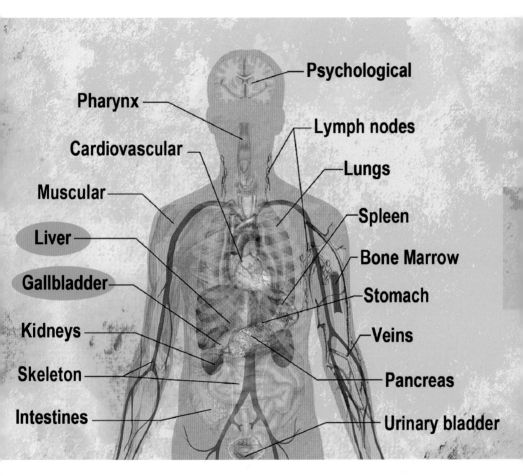

- Psychological
- Pharynx
- Lymph nodes
- Cardiovascular
- Lungs
- Muscular
- Spleen
- Liver
- Bone Marrow
- Gallbladder
- Stomach
- Kidneys
- Veins
- Skeleton
- Pancreas
- Intestines
- Urinary bladder

When the liver is out of balance, there is a blockage of energy and in the flow of fluids. Tendons are not moistened and can easily tear, become inflamed, or cause unusual contraction or weakness in their related muscles. A common result of liver stagnation is an inflexible and rigid body.

Paired Organ of Wood

The hollow organ that is paired with
the liver is the gallbladder.

Liver — Stomach
Duodenum — Gall Bladder
Pancreas — Spleen
Ascending Colon — Transverse Colon
Small Intestine — Large Intestine
Appendix — Rectum
— Anus

The gallbladder stores about 2 ounces of bile, which is released when food containing fat enters the digestive tract. The bile emulsifies fats and neutralizes acids in partly digested food. Bile is made of 3 parts. One is bile salt made from cholesterol, one is a pigment from dead red blood cells that give stool a brownish color, and another is waste and toxins.

The condition of the gallbladder is dependent on our intake of fats and oils. Americans eat 300 pounds of dairy products and 200 pounds of meat a year, plus 35 pounds of oils. These fats can solidify in the gallbladder and create stones.

If the gallbladder has been removed, it can't store bile and the liver must work harder from then on. You can live fine but need to limit fat and consume more sour foods.

Cold drinks can solidify fats in the gallbladder. We drink about 1.5 quarts of 40-degree liquids a day.

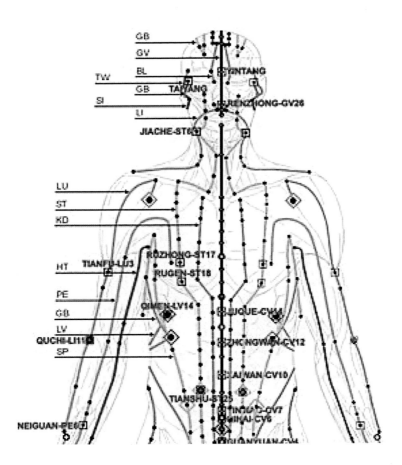

Body Part Association

Each organ is associated with, or considered to rule, a certain body part and sense organ.

Liver rules the ligaments and tendons.
It has a relation to the shoulders.

The liver meridian passes through the eyes. Cataracts, glaucoma, red or dry eyes, night blindness, excessive tearing, far- and nearsightedness, and other eye conditions reflect the condition of the liver.

Sense Organ Association

The liver corresponds to the eyes

- If the whites of the eyes look yellowish or get crusty (or regular visits from the sandman) in the morning, the cause is fat accumulation in the liver.

- If eyes are red or bloodshot or if you get red spots or styes on the eyes, lids, or between the eyes, it's due to a swollen and inflamed liver.

- If eyes are watery or swollen or burn or itch, it's from a swollen liver. Dryness is an overly contracted condition.

I have seen many eye conditions cleared up merely by addressing the liver and not even treating the eyes directly.

I have found that sudden bloody spots on the whites of the eyes often happen after eating a combination of too much fat with sweet, like icecream or chocolate.

The Taste of Wood
The flavor associated with the liver and gallbladder is sour

Sour flavor has a dispersing effect on the liver, so this is good if the liver is tight and full of fat. To help the liver deal with fat and oil add more green vegetables like broccoli, collards, scallions.

If you wake up grouchy, it's due to liver stagnation. When wood energy is flowing smoothly you have patience. If you're tense and irritable and angry at traffic, you may need to eat less oil and saturated fat.

Fermented vegetables are a good source for the sour flavor. Vegetable juices can also reduce excess in the liver, especially with greens. So add celery, kale or parsley to your carrot juice.

The sour flavor can help with abnormal leakage of fluid or energy such as urinary dripping, excess perspiration, hemorrhage, and diarrhea. It can also firm up tissues in cases such as flaccid skin, hemorrhoids and uterine prolapse.

63

Nourishing Wood

Examples of wood nourishing foods are:

- Tomato
- Barley
- Vinegar
- Pickles
- Sauerkraut
- Green apples
- Lemons
- Grapefruit

Besides increasing raw foods in spring, use a shorter cooking time but at a higher temperature, so the food is not thoroughly cooked, especially the inner part.

When using water use light steaming or minimal simmering.

If using oil, a quick high temperature sauté method is best.

Wood Cooking Styles

Wood cooking styles include:
pickling, blanching, pressed salad
or steaming. Grilling, smoking and
steaming are also associated with the
wood element.

For a pressed salad, massage shredded
vegetables with salt, then put them
in a pickle press or put a plate over
the veggies with a weight on top until
water comes out of the vegetables.
You can try this with lettuce, radishes,
cucumbers, or spinach, and press for
about 24 hours.

Liver/Gallbladder and Oils

Bile made in the liver is stored in the gallbladder, which secretes it into the small intestine to emulsify and digest oils.

Avoid low-quality oils such as cottonseed, canola, corn, and soy. The best oils are olive, coconut, sesame and grapeseed.

Herbs for Liver

Dandelion is an overall liver cleanser and tonic. It is particularly effective for premenstrual mood swings accompanied by bloating and breast tenderness.

Peppermint is a mood-elevating, invigorating herb that also helps with digestive disturbances, bloating, and poor appetite. Take as a tea and drink freely throughout the day.

Burdock root cleanses the liver and blood, can be cooked when fresh, like a carrot, or used in a tea when dried.

Milk thistle is the premier herb for anyone who has been exposed to toxic chemicals. It should be taken for at least 2 months after exposure. It is beneficial for people who work with chemicals or are routinely exposed to pollution.

Cheladonium is one of the best overall liver tonics. It should be taken as a tincture -- a few drops in a tablespoon of water -- 3 times a day before meals, and it will quickly clear digestive and appetite disturbances, enhance clarity of vision, and ease emotional strain.

The Liver and Emotions

Planning ability and good judgment are marks of a healthy liver.

Emotions related to anger are one of the first signs of a liver imbalance: impatience, frustration, resentment, violence, belligerence, rudeness, arrogance, stubbornness, aggression, and an impulsive or explosive personality. If these are repressed, they can cause depression.

The gallbladder is small, so little angers like frustration and irritability can show up. Mood swings and emotional excesses in general are liver-related.

A healthy liver ensures patience, alertness, endurance, perseverance, the energetic pursuit of spiritual development, and the maintenance of a strong spiritual center.

Photograph: Stuart Pilbrow http://bit.ly/12P1w6

The Spirit of Liver

The Spirit that incarnates in the liver is called the Hun. It has to do with vision, imagination, dreams, direction, decision, and justice. It also has to do with benevolence and finding one's true path.

As you work with and heal your liver, the home for the Hun, you should achieve...

- More clarity and direction in your life purpose

- Increased ability to achieve your goals with less procrastination

- Better imagination and guidance through day and night dreams

- More emotional stability with the ability to know what you're feeling and stand by your feelings and beliefs

- Less indecisiveness, guilt, timidity, irritability and depression

- More passion and excitement in life with zest and a more colorful life

- Less blaming of others and feeling that life is unfair

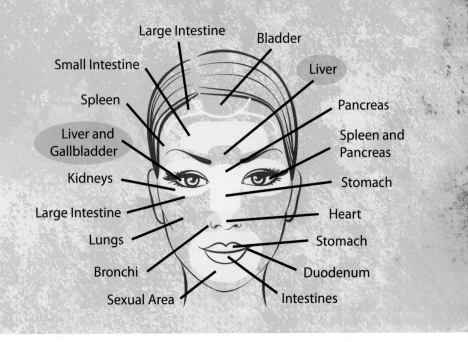

Large Intestine
Bladder
Small Intestine
Liver
Spleen
Pancreas
Liver and
Gallbladder
Spleen and
Pancreas
Kidneys
Stomach
Large Intestine
Heart
Lungs
Stomach
Bronchi
Duodenum
Sexual Area
Intestines

Facial Diagnosis

- **The face never lies.**

- The area between the eyebrows indicates the state of the liver.

- The gallbladder is outside that area and near the hairline at the edges of forehead.

In general, redness or puffiness is related to yin or expansive energy. This can be from sugar or excess sweets, citrus, chemicals, spices, vinegar, or alcohol. Tightness or darker colors can be from too much yang or contractive energy, perhaps from too much meat, eggs, cheese, or salt. White colorations can be from many milk products.

A deep line between the eyebrows means the liver is overly contracted. If there are several shallow vertical lines the liver is overly expanded.

Remember that the color of the wood element is green, so a greenish complexion or patches can relate to liver or gallbladder, but also can be a precancerous sign.

The Liver Meridian

- From the inside of the big toe, up inner leg to groin to under breast.

- 14 acupuncture points.

- The liver stores the blood and is responsible for maintaining the free flow of Qi throughout the body.

- The liver can affect digestion, menstruation, tendons and ligaments, bile production, and eye problems.

Some problems related to the liver meridian: uterus or prostate problems, genital problems, inner knee and thigh pain or skin issues or varicose veins, big toe problems like gout or nail fungus, or ingrown toenail.

Besides traversing just below the surface of the skin, meridians also dive deeper into the body in an internal pathway.

In addition to the meridian flow along the skin, there are deeper internal pathways. Problems with the internal pathways can cause diaphragm and lung conditions, tightness in the chest, the feeling of something in the throat (plum pit) and eye pain.

LR 14
LR 13
LR 12
LR 11
LR 10
LR 9
LR 8
LR 7
LR 6
LR 5
LR 4
LR 3
LR 2
LR 1

71

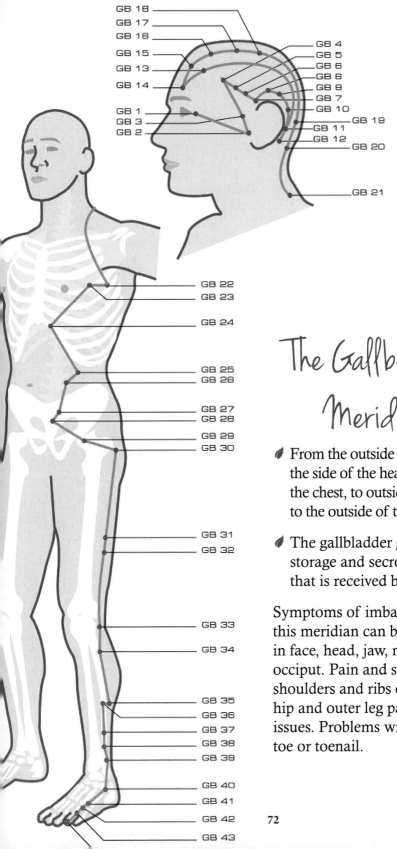

GB 18
GB 17
GB 16
GB 15
GB 13
GB 14
GB 1
GB 3
GB 2
GB 4
GB 5
GB 6
GB 8
GB 9
GB 7
GB 10
GB 19
GB 11
GB 12
GB 20
GB 21

GB 22
GB 23
GB 24
GB 25
GB 26
GB 27
GB 28
GB 29
GB 30
GB 31
GB 32
GB 33
GB 34
GB 35
GB 36
GB 37
GB 38
GB 39
GB 40
GB 41
GB 42
GB 43

The Gallbladder Meridian

- From the outside of the eyes, the side of the head, the side of the chest, to outside of the leg, to the outside of the 4th toe.

- The gallbladder governs the storage and secretion of bile that is received by the liver.

Symptoms of imbalance with this meridian can be pain in face, head, jaw, neck, or occiput. Pain and stiffness of shoulders and ribs or shingles, hip and outer leg pain or skin issues. Problems with the 4th toe or toenail.

72

Acu Point for Liver

Liver 3-Taichong-Supreme Rushing

Location: Slide your finger up between the 2nd and big toe on top of the foot, in the valley where the bones come together.

Benefits: Helps the liver, good for migraines, menstrual problems, digestive disorders, irritability, insomnia, dizziness, exhaustion, and headaches.

For stress, tension and to clear the head, treat this point along with Large Intestine 4, called the Four Gates.

For acupressure, use your middle or index finger at a 90-degree angle to the points. Apply firm and steady pressure. This may be tender but shouldn't be painful. Hold the point for about 3 minutes. You can also visualize light coming out of your finger and illuminating the meridian and the associated organ.

Gallbladder Acu Point

Gallbladder 41-Zulingqi-Foot Near to Tears

Location: On the top side of the foot, slide up 1 inch between the 4th and 5th toes, in the groove between the bones.

Benefits: Hip pain, shoulder tension, moving joint pains, headaches, dizziness, side aches, water retention, sciatic and foot pain.

Time of Day Wood Meridians Peak

Energy peaks in the liver channel at 11 PM to 1 AM.

Energy peaks in the gallbladder channel at 1 AM to 3 AM.

Healing Sound for Liver

Qigong has a healing sound for the major organs.

Xu (pronounced *shu-yii*)

STEP 1: Stand naturally. Overlap your hands on top of your abdomen. Men: place your left hand a few finger spaces below the navel. Women: place your right hand on the same area.

STEP 2: Inhale. Imagine leading energy from your right big toe up the inside of your right leg past the reproductive organs, up below your right rib cage and up just below your right breast.

STEP 3: Exhale. Open your eyes wide and mentally look into your liver. Let out the *Xu* (Shuuu-yiii) sound as you lean forward slightly. At the same time, hold up the center of your perineum and draw your abdomen in to squeeze out the impurities from your liver. Repeat for 6 inhalations and exhalations.

The Water Element
The Kidney and Bladder

Water

After such hard work, enjoy a shower
Though I am soft, I have no less power

My drops, through eons erode any rock
My nebulous vapor can rust any lock

I seek all places deep and low
I run not or jump, I relax and flow

I am the moist eyes of every daughter
To life I am mother, they know me as water

Lakes and oceans, rainstorm and dew
After the drought, all life I renew

Steam me, I'll condense, freeze me, I'll melt
I'm the flow of emotion, can't be known, just felt

I clean out all toxins, remove all debris
No one can live a moment without me

Hear me in song in the cry of the loon
Poets depict me in the face of the moon

Restrict my expression and soon you'll be old
Life is for living, water you can't hold

I love to dance in fountain and spring
In each beating heart, in each cell do I sing

My essence can fill the deepest hole
Feel now my presence thou precious soul.

—Warren King

Energy of Water

Imagine as water goes from ice
to flowing liquid water
before it vaporizes.

It has no form of its own and follows
the course of least resistance.

It seems weak, but it can carve the deepest
canyon and wear down the hardest rock.

Water in the Daily Cycle

◊ Water corresponds to nighttime

◊ The time after sunset (metal) and before sunrise (wood)

How is your night?

Night shift is called the graveyard shift for a reason, kidneys recharge at night so being awake at that time makes it hard to recharge your batteries.

Nighttime problems like insomnia or night sweats may be kidney related. So would tossing and turning in bed, grinding teeth at night, nightmares, bed wetting or waking at night to urinate.

Water in the Yearly Cycle

Water is connected with the winter

Nature goes within during winter

Winter is like the nighttime of the year

Winter is cold, not much is happening. Movement is slow, quiet and still. Plants send their energy to the roots, animals slow down and some hibernate.

Kidneys like warmth and heat, so cold extremities are a sign of weak kidneys. Use of a ginger compress is a home remedy for weak kidneys. Sauna may benefit them as well.

Water Element Organs

Water corresponds to the solid organ of the kidneys.

Each kidney is about 5 inches long and 3 inches wide. One of the main jobs is to filter waste out of your 1 to 1.5 gallons of blood as many as 400 times a day!

The kidneys also balance the volume of fluids and minerals in the body. They even make some of their own hormones, such as the one that tells the body to make red blood cells. The kidneys can also help regulate blood pressure.

The adrenal glands are associated with the kidneys and help protect against mental stress. In Chinese medicine kidneys are viewed as the center of the vital force or chi so it's important to keep them strong. They enable us to go out into life and handle problems.

- Salt can tighten kidneys and make them hold water. Too much protein can be hard on the kidneys. Meat is often a cause of kidney stones. Men need more protein than women and women need more oil than men.

- The average person eats 9 pounds of chemicals a year, a big stress on kidneys. Heavy metals such as mercury in silver fillings are an additional stressor.

- Kidneys are often the underlying cause of arthritis.

- Soft drinks high in phosphoric acid and sugar are hard on kidneys.

- Kidneys rule sexual energy, so people on Viagra® and similar drugs really need to strengthen the kidneys.

- If the kidneys are hard or calloused there can be fatty deposits or stones in the kidneys.

- Kidneys can affect posture. Leaning forward can mean kidneys are too tight, and leaning backward when walking, sitting, and standing can indicate overly expanded kidneys.

Paired Organ of the Kidneys is Bladder

The hollow paired organ of the kidney is the urinary bladder.

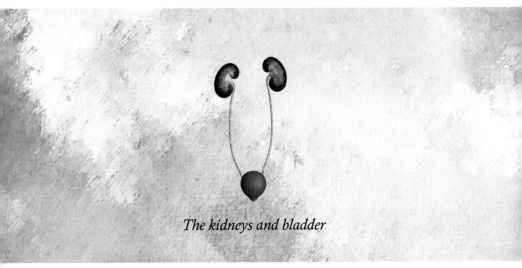

The kidneys and bladder

The bladder is a storage sac that holds the urine. When the bladder is about halfway full, your body tells you to urinate.

The bladder is such a simple organ that scientists are beginning to be able to grow them in a lab.

Your Constitution

It is thought that our inherited energy, or Jing, is stored in our kidneys. **It is like a battery that we run on for the rest of our life, and it is not easy to recharge it once it has run down.**

Your constitution is what you are born with. But your condition is how you are now. So if you are born with a strong constitution but sleep little, play hard, take drugs, smoke or use alcohol excessively, eat too much, or are consumed with worry and frustration, you could have a shorter life. Likewise, if you inherited a weak constitution, but eat very cleanly, sleep long enough, exercise and meditate, you could have a longer life.

Those with stronger constitutions are like hardwood; they can handle more wear and tear and more stress. Those who are weaker, like softwood, show every bump and scratch. They need more rest and sleep and can't push themselves too far or hard.

- A stronger or yang constitution can be seen in having stronger and bigger bones.

- A large head to body ratio is yang; 1:7 is balanced, 1:6 more yang, 1:8 more yin. So taller people tend to be more yin and shorter more yang.

- A longer face is more yin and a more square face is more yang.

Ears reflect the kidneys which are associated with inherited energy. If they are larger, thicker, lower set, flatter against the head, and larger lobed, then they are more yang.

Body Part Association

Each organ is associated with, or considered to rule, a certain body part and sense organ. **Kidneys rule the bones and joints**, especially the knees and ankles, and may contribute to arthritis because they flush out calcium and other minerals in the urine.

Kidneys have to do with the spine, and particularly the lower back.

If you break bones easily, then you likely have weak kidneys. Osteoporosis and osteopenia are related to weak kidneys, like you are urinating out your minerals instead of keeping them in place. Depositing minerals in the wrong places, as in kidney stones or in joints contributing to arthritis, is a kidney issue. Low back pain is often due to weak kidneys.

Sense Organ Association

The kidneys correspond to the ears.

It is interesting how our ears are shaped like kidneys. There is a map, actually 3 maps, on the ear that let you treat and diagnose the entire body, as in reflexology. One kidney point is right where the earring hole typically is. A big ear and earlobe is a sign of strong kidneys and thus a long life; look at the earlobes on a Buddha statue! Very old people often have large earlobes. Hearing loss or ringing in the ears is a sign of weak kidneys.

The Taste of Water

The flavor associated with the kidneys and bladder is salty.

Salt is not necessarily good for the kidneys, but it is involved with the kidneys. The World Health Organization advised having 1/5 the salt found in the Standard American Diet.

Good salt choices: Himalayan or Celtic sea salt, soy sauce, miso (best used in cooking, not raw on food), and gomashio, a sesame salt combination. The sesame oil coats the salt so it gets into cells.

- To grains and vegetables, add a pinch of salt to bring out sweetness. If food tastes salty, you added too much.

- Sea salt has 10% magnesium which calms stress. Table salt has none.

- Sea vegetables are high in trace minerals. Have them in a side dish of 1—3 tsp a day.

- Salt should be greatly reduced for those with damp, overweight, lethargic, or edema conditions and for those with high blood pressure.

- Salt has a cooling effect and moves energy downward and inward. It softens hardened lumps and stiffness and improves digestion, detoxifies the body and can purge the bowels.

- If you eat salt by itself, you'll crave water or sweet.

Salt can be used in heat conditions such as gargling for a sore throat, brushed with for bleeding gums, or used in a neti pot for inflamed sinuses. It increases appetite and is thus misused in the form of common table salt, which is of poor quality.

Nourishing Water Foods

Examples of foods that nourish kidneys and bladder are:

- ◆ Tofu
- ◆ Miso
- ◆ Eggs
- ◆ Fish
- ◆ Soy sauce
- ◆ Burdock root
- ◆ Seaweed vegetables (wakame, kombu, arame, hiziki, kelp, nori, and dulce)

Even though many people should cut back on salt, seaweed is fine to eat. Its iodine and trace minerals actually speed up metabolism.

Much of our soil has been depleted of trace minerals. Seaweeds have all these minerals and a secret missing ingredient in the health of the kidneys. It is said that nori, the wrapper for sushi, is especially good for a weak bladder. Miso soup is an excellent kidney tonic.

Water Cooking Styles

Water cooking styles include stewing, frying, and nabe (a covered shallow ceramic Japanese pot).

Eater is associated with winter. So as salads are great for spring and summer, in the winter, to keep warm and nourish our kidneys we need more stews, which are, of course, watery and you can have more salt than in the warmer seasons.

Frying in oil gives us more calories and fat so we can keep warm in the winter. It is harder for the body to lose weight in the winter because it is in a food-storage mode.

Kidney/Bladder and Salt

Even though most people abuse low-quality salt and suffer for it, good-quality salt is essential for the health of every cell.

Avoid commercial salt. Instead get sea salt, Celtic sea salt is very healthy, as is Himalayan salt. Both have many trace minerals.

Other good sources of salt are miso, tamari, soy sauce, umeboshi plums (pictured), and sea vegetables.

Since salt is very yang and contracting, if eaten in excess it can cause tightness in the body and make one feel too tense.

Herbs for Kidneys and Bladder

Corn silk

Gotu kola

Juniper berries

Parsley

Uva ursi

Red clover

Stinging nettle tea

Black tea

The Kidneys and Emotions

- The kidneys are associated with will, memory and confidence.

- Imbalanced kidney energy produces a lack of will, action and direction.

- Fear and anxiety indicate weak kidneys.

If the kidneys are out of balance, you can feel afraid, overwhelmed, confused, and lack confidence. **When in balance, you feel courageous, you know your own mind and feel self-confident and are committed and action-oriented.**

Kidney energy has to do with our drive or will in life, including our degree of aggression, sex drive, courage, and follow-through, endurance, and right timing.

If the kidneys are too tired, one can be overly aggressive or violent, stubborn, moving too fast or insensitive to the space and rhythm of others, often with attachment to the past.

If too tired and swollen, one can be passive, lazy, fearful, lose concern for time, procrastinate or arrive late, lack courage and ambition, and lose appetite for sex or life in general.

The Spirit of the Kidneys

- The Spirit that incarnates in the kidneys is called the Zhi.

- Psychologically Zhi has to do with instinctual power and is aligned with will and courage.

- Forgetfulness, lack of motivation, addiction, depression, fear, sexual issues, sleep disturbance and controlling others can be signs of an imbalanced Zhi.

Affecting the Zhi...

- Any time the will is employed to push the body beyond its own limits; overwork, excessive physical activity, such as excess marathon running, biking, weight lifting

- Use of substances that impinge on adrenal function, such as caffeine, amphetamines, steroids, or cortisone, and chronic disease

- Addictive behavior of any kind, including excess sexual activity, chronic fear and anxiety, particularly during childhood, shock, trauma, and guilt

- Multiple births and excess blood loss during periods

- A lack of discipline and encouragement during childhood

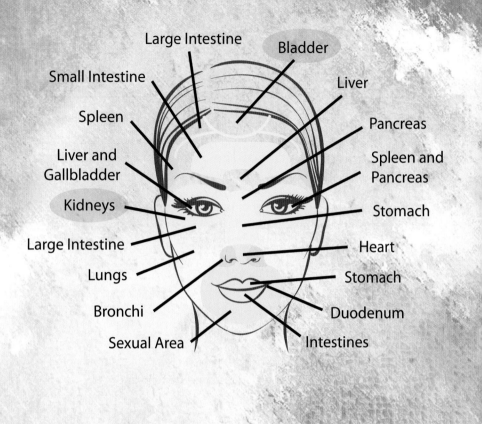

Large Intestine
Bladder
Small Intestine
Liver
Spleen
Pancreas
Liver and Gallbladder
Spleen and Pancreas
Kidneys
Stomach
Large Intestine
Heart
Lungs
Stomach
Bronchi
Duodenum
Sexual Area
Intestines

Facial Diagnosis

- **The face never lies.**

- The area below the eyes tells the state of the kidneys.

- The chin can also reflect the kidneys and bladder.

Dark or black under the eyes denotes toxic blood due to inadequate detoxification by the kidneys. If skin is drawn and tight under eyes it's a contracted condition. If puffy and swollen it's expanded kidneys. Interestingly, we think of people with a large chin to have more will and a receding chin as being weak willed. This has to do with the inherited kidney energy, which also rules sexuality. A cleft chin is even more contracted or yang, indicating more power.

The Kidney Meridian

♦ From bottom of foot, around ankle, up inner leg to below the clavicle.

♦ 27 acupuncture points.

♦ The kidney is responsible for fluid metabolism and the storage of Jing (essence).

♦ The kidney affects reproduction, teeth, bones, water metabolism, hair loss, and sexual energy.

Meridian can affect lungs, ears, breast, solar plexus, digestion, bladder, and reproductive organs.

Pain, weakness, or skin issues along the meridian, and pain behind the knee and lumbar vertebrae, sacrum and coccyx, as well as pain or skin issues or fungus on soles of feet.

The Bladder Meridian

BL 6
BL 5
BL 4
BL 3
BL 2
BL 1

BL 4
BL 5
BL 6
BL 7

BL 8
BL 9
BL 10

BL 11
BL 12
BL 13
BL 14
BL 15
BL 16
BL 17
BL 18
BL 19
BL 20
BL 21
BL 22
BL 23
BL 24
BL 25
BL 26
BL 27
BL 28
BL 29
BL 30
BL 35

BL 36
BL 37
BL 38
BL 39
BL 40
BL 41
BL 42
BL 43
BL 44
BL 45
BL 46
BL 47
BL 48
BL 49
BL 50
BL 51
BL 52
BL 53
BL 54
BL 55
BL 56
BL 57
BL 58
BL 59
BL 60
BL 61
BL 62
BL 63
BL 64
BL 65
BL 66
BL 67

◆ From inside of the eyes, over scalp, along 2 lines on the sides of the spine, down back of leg to outside of pinky toe.

◆ 67 acupuncture points.

◆ The bladder has to do with the excretion of urine.

Meridian issues can be hair loss, headaches, sinus, and eye problems. Spine pain or stiffness. Low back pain and sciatica, calf pain, and weak ankles or feet. Pinky toe is the end of the channel. Research has shown that heating the end point on the outer corner of the pinky nail can turn a breach baby.

Acu Point for the Kidney

Kidney 3-taixi-Great Mountain Stream

Location: Midway between inner ankle bone and the Achilles tendon.

Benefits: Tatigue, menstrual irregularities, impotence, low back pain, headache, sore throat, toothache, hearing loss, ringing in the ears, insomnia, swollen feet, ankle pain.

For acupressure, use your middle or index finger at a 90-degree angle to the points. Apply firm and steady pressure. It may be tender but shouldn't be painful. Hold the point for about 3 minutes. You can also visualize light coming out of your finger and illuminating the meridian and the associated organ.

Bladder Acu Point

Bladder 60-Kun Lun-Kunlun Mountain

Location: Midway between the outer ankle bone and the achilles tendon.

Benefits: Main point for any spine pain, low back pain, pain or numbness in lower limbs, good for excess type headaches where there is too much energy that is stagnant.

Time of Day Water Meridians Peak

Energy peaks in the bladder channel at 3 PM to 5 PM.

Energy peaks in the kidney channel at 5 PM to 7 PM.

If you have an energy drop in the late afternoon, it could indicate a blockage of these organ and meridian. Sometimes you may notice that if you exercise at this time, you have another burst of energy and you won't feel like napping.

Healing Sound for the Kidneys

Qigong has a healing sound for the major organs.
Chui (*Chew-eee*) is the sound for the kidneys.

STEP 1: Stand (or sit) with your feet shoulder width apart, arms to your sides. Inhale and raise your hands up towards your lower back with the back of your hands facing your body. As your hands reach kidney level, bring both hands forward towards your belly button with fingers pointing down. As you raise your hands, lead energy up from the bottom of your right foot along the inside of your right leg into the tailbone and along the lower part of your spine into your kidneys. Continue the arm movements and bring your arms in front of your chest until they are right below your collar bone, then turn your palms to face each other. Exhale. Make the *Chui* (*Chew-eee*) sound by opening your mouth slightly with your tongue drawn in and the corner of your mouth pulled slightly to the sides. At the same time, squeeze in with your hands as though you were holding a ball, then squat down.

STEP 2: Keep your upper body as straight as you can. Hold up the center of the perineum and pull your abdomen in. As you exhale and make the *Chui* sound, imagine leading all impurities from your kidneys out of your mouth.

STEP 3: Stand up slowly and repeat Steps 1—2 a total of six times.

Taking Care of Water

- Nourishing food, rest, meditation, and natural beauty

- Calming physical exercise, such as yoga, tai chi and qigong

- Avoidance of excess thinking, working, and craving; maintaining a reasonable schedule and making special time each day to do nothing

- Spend time with water, get a foot massage, use guided imagery and practice meditation

As you strengthen your kidneys you will feel empowered instead of drained by life.

Other changes may include:

- A sense of power and equilibrium

- Increased serenity as you stop trying to control the world around you

- An increased sense of trust

- The ability to know and speak your authentic feelings and to stay with projects until they are complete

- Less fear and anxiety, more excitement and curiosity, courage to face the unknown

- Developing a definite sense of what matters to you, increased initiative, motivation, and perseverance

- You will be regarded by others as someone to trust

The Fire Element
Heart and
Small Intestine

Fire

I am the fire of the Central Sun
The light of life, of everyone

The heat that keeps the bloodstream warm
The lightning of the thunderstorm

Wisdom of the sage's mind
All impure I shall refine

Bees buzzing on a summer day
Children jumping, as they laugh and play

Quasars, pulsars, electrons, too
All that's old I shall renew

The hearth that comforts every home
I breathe in every centrosome

The glint in every warrior's eye
The faith that martyrs never die

The glow of cosmos, the light of space
The speed of thought, desire to race

Beyond all form and every name
Behold, I beat thine own heart flame.

—Warren King

Energy of Fire

Fire is the most expansive energy.

It is upward and outward.

Flames are always moving upward.

It is a more extreme energy that occurs between wood energy, which is gently moving upward, and earth energy, which is beginning to settle.

Fire in the Daily Cycle

＊ Since fire is the most upward energy, it has to do with the time when the sun is highest in the sky.

＊ So fire energy peaks around noon.

＊ We are most awake at that time.

Fire in the Yearly Cycle

＊ Summer is like the noontime of the year.

＊ Fire moves upward and outward.

＊ There is a literal buzzing energy in summer; the crickets, cicadas, birds, and frogs are singing.

Most people love summer. Everything is blossoming, nature is noisy and bustling with energy. People often take time off from school and work and play more and spend time outside, although sometimes it can get too hot. We don't want to cook very much in a hot kitchen.

Fire Element Organs

Fire corresponds to the heart

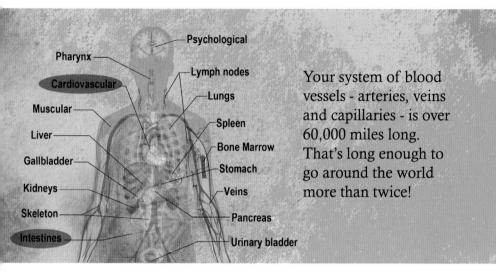

Psychological
Pharynx
Cardiovascular
Muscular
Liver
Gallbladder
Kidneys
Skeleton
Intestines

Lymph nodes
Lungs
Spleen
Bone Marrow
Stomach
Veins
Pancreas
Urinary bladder

Your system of blood vessels - arteries, veins and capillaries - is over 60,000 miles long. That's long enough to go around the world more than twice!

* The adult heart pumps about 5 quarts of blood each minute, approximately 2,000 gallons of blood each day throughout the body. That's 400 5 gallon bottles.

* The heart beats about 100,000 times each day. In a 70-year lifetime, the average human heart beats more than 2.5 billion times.

* A child's heart is about the size of a clenched fist; an adult's heart is about the size of 2 fists.

* Blood takes about 20 seconds to circulate throughout the entire vascular system.

* Expansive foods weaken the heart: alcohol, coffee, caffeine. They are yin, and can cause the heart to swell and beat irregularly. A fatty, compacted heart is a more yang condition. If you eat the Standard American Diet for 30 to 60 years you will get blockages from hard fats, meats, eggs, and cheese.

Paired Organ of Fire

The hollow organ paired with the heart is the small intestine.

* The small intestine is about 23 feet long and 1.5 inches wide. About 90% of what we eat is assimilated (enters the blood) in the small intestine.

* Food is alkalized in the small intestine with the help of enzymes secreted from the pancreas and gallbladder. It has a huge surface area, 10 times greater than the skin, with folds and villi (finger-like projections) with smaller villi on them.

* Food goes from the small intestine to the liver via the portal vein, but fat goes directly into the lymphatic system. Leaky gut is a very common and serious problem. When the tight junctions between the cells break down and the villi become permeable, then whole molecules of proteins can get into the bloodstream. The body perceives these as being invaders and launches an immune response and you can end up with a food allergy. Worse than that is the fact that these antibodies can then target the body's own cells, which are similar to the foods. So instead of just attacking the wheat gluten molecule, the immune system can attack your own pancreas cells and create diabetes.

Body Part Association

Each organ is associated with, or considered to rule, a certain body part and sense organ. **Heart rules the blood vessels.**

So varicose veins or bruising easily may indicate a problem with the heart energy.

ography: Patrick J. Lynch, medical illustrator http://bit.ly/1cN1G

Sense Organ Association

The heart corresponds to the tongue (called the sprout of the heart).

A sore on your tongue may indicate heat in the heart meridian. Stuttering or stammering in speech can indicate a heart murmur or hyperactive heartbeat. These can also lead to jerky kinds of movements, or the inability to sit still or get comfortable.

The Taste of Fire

The flavor associated with the heart
and small intestine is bitter.

Bitter is mostly missing from the American
diet, except for coffee and chocolate. A
better choice would be bitter greens like
arugula or sesame seeds.

Isn't it interesting that we have very little
bitter flavor in our diets, and heart disease
is the number one cause of death.

Photograph: Barny achmad http://bit.ly/19NgZNS

Nourishing Fire

Bitter is eaten in the least quantity of all the 5 tastes but we should have it regularly.

- Kale
- Dandelion
- Arugula
- Sesame seeds
- Bitter greens
- Daikon radish
- Brussel sprouts
- Celery
- Lettuce
- Broccoli
- Endive
- Collard greens
- Quinoa
- Orange peel
- Kumquats
- Black currants

- **Shiitake mushroom** help clear cholesterol from blood vessels. Cholesterol sticks more if the blood vessels are damaged by high sugar in the blood.

- The heart likes a rhythmic life: regular sleeping, waking, and eating times.

- A fatty meal makes platelets stick together like sludge for 6 hours, then another meal is eaten so the blood never flows well. All organs and cells depend on good circulation.

- Bitter helps to lower blood pressure, and **celery** is specifically good for this. Bitter is said to drain dampness, so it is good for Candida yeast overgrowth, parasites, mucus, skin eruptions, tumors, cysts, edema, and obesity.

- Bitter foods are especially good for those who are slow, overweight, lethargic and damp or watery, and also good for overheated and aggressive people. On the other hand, those who are thin, cold, weak and nervous should limit bitter.

Fire Cooking Styles

* Food preparations include: raw, pressed salad, stir frying and blanching, as well as toasting and dehydration. Appetizers and snacks are also ruled by the fire element.

* Besides increasing raw foods in spring, when cooking, it should be with a shorter cooking time but at a higher temperature, so the food is not cooked through, especially the inner part.

* When using water, use light steaming or minimal simmering. If you use oil then a quick high temperature sauté method is best.

Heart and Exercise

* People with an active lifestyle have 45% less heart disease than sedentary people.

* Sedentary people have a 35% higher incidence of high blood pressure than active people.

* Exercise helps cholesterol levels and reduces inflammation in the arteries.

* It is recommended to get 150 minutes of moderate, or 75 minutes of vigorous exercise a week.

Herbs for Heart

* Hawthorne
* Capsicum/Cayenne
* Chickweed
* Garlic
* Olive leaf
* Hawthorn
* Lavender
* Green tea
* Oregano
* Cayenne
* Chickweed
* Olive leaf

The Heart and Emotions

Joy is the emotion of the heart when balanced.

An imbalanced heart can result in:

* Panic or hysteria.

* Some psychological difficulties involving defective self-image.

* Problems with relationships in general.

The heart is like the central headquarters for incoming information from the other organs. With a heart out of balance, a person can be overexcited, too tense, unable to enjoy life, or a workaholic. **When balanced you feel more relaxed, playful, lighter, inspired, and celebratory.**

The Spirit of the Heart

* The Spirit that incarnates in the heart is called the Shen.

* It is the fiery spark of consciousness and is reflected in the light shining from the eyes.

* Its virtues are compassion and love.

* Sleeping problems and disturbed dreams are Shen imbalances.

Photograph: ©2015 Connie Hoskin Art

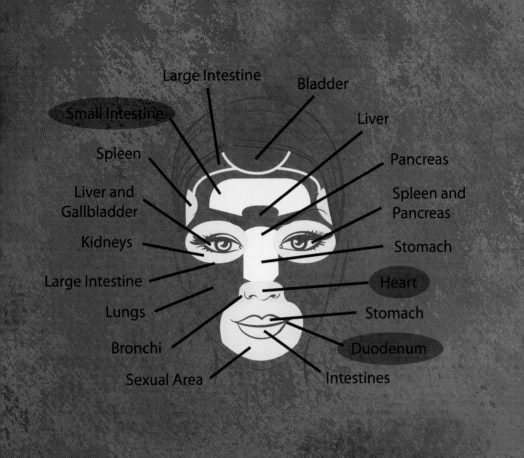

Facial Diagnosis

* **The face never lies.**

* The nose represents the state of the heart.

* The small intestine can be reflected in the corners of the mouth and inside of the lips as well as the middle of the forehead.

Facial Diagnosis

A swollen or reddish face may mean a heart issue, with redness indicating high blood pressure, especially if there are expanded capillaries of the nose.

Purple on the tip of the nose indicates that the heart is weak and has lost much of its elasticity and strength, and may mean low blood pressure, a more advanced condition than if red.

Waxy pallor on some noses are fat deposits surrounding the heart, usually too much saturated fat in the diet. Herbs like ginger, scallions, garlic, and daikon radish can melt away these fat deposits.

When you have cracks or sores on the corners of the mouth, it usually indicates poor food combinations, as do sores on the inside of your lips. Sometimes we bite our lips when chewing, that is usually due to an inflammation of the inside of the lips, which reflects an inflamed small intestine.

Balance

Shen (spirit) imbalances are:

- Anxiety
- Palpitations
- Difficulty concentrating
- Being timid or easily startled
- Being overly talkative - remember that the heart rules the tongue
- Mania or schizophrenia
- Being incoherent in speech
- Being hyperactive and restless

A person with a balanced Shen:

- Unique individual with a unique path
- Has self-reflection and can distinguish the true from the unreal

Anything that upsets the heart upsets the Shen. Emotional trauma, shock, and abuse can cause a Shen disturbance, as can recreational drugs and excessive alcohol.

The Heart Meridian

❊ From underarm to inside of the pinky finger.

❊ 9 acupuncture points.

❊ The heart governs the circulation of blood and is the residence of Shen (spirit) and has to do with clear thinking.

❊ Shen disturbance may manifest as insomnia, excess dreaming, or forgetfulness. A more seriously imbalanced condition may include hysteria, irrational behavior, insanity, or delirium.

Other disorders may include palpitations or skipped beats, rapid heartbeat, chest pain, and heart disorders.

A meridian disorder can give numbness, stiffness, or pain along the inner arm or the pinky finger or nail. Pain or swollen glands in the armpit can be heart related.

SI 19
SI 18
SI 17
SI 16
SI 15
SI 14
SI 13
SI 12
SI 10
SI 9
SI 11
SI 8
SI 7
SI 6
SI 5
SI 4
SI 3
SI 2
SI 1

Small Intestine Meridian

* From outside of the pinky finger to scapula to in front of the ear.

* 21 acupuncture points.

* Receives food from the stomach.

* Separates nutrition from waste.

The small intestine meridian goes to the ears and face, so hearing loss or facial neuralgia may be signs of imbalance. Also swollen lymph nodes in the throat and scapula or shoulder pain or skin issues along the meridian to the outer pinky.

I used to get pain on my outer pinky nail if I had eaten bad food combinations.

119

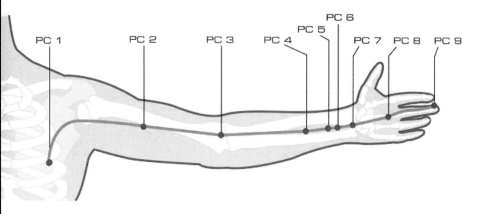

PC 1 PC 2 PC 3 PC 4 PC 5 PC 6 PC 7 PC 8 PC 9

Pericardium Meridian

* The pericardium is called the "heart protector."

* It is also considered a fire element organ.

* If the heart is the "Emperor," then the pericardium is the "Ambassador."

* It is the first line of defense protecting the heart from external pathogenic influence.

* Often the heart is treated in acupuncture not directly but through the pericardium meridian.

* 9 points, starting near the nipples down inside of the arm to tip of the middle finger.

Triple Warmer Meridian

* The only meridian that has no corresponding physical organ.

* It is paired with the pericardium and is also considered part of the fire element.

* It consist of 3 warmers: upper in chest, middle in stomach area, and lower in lower abdomen.

* It has to do with metabolism and digestion.

* From the ring finger, up the middle of outside of the arm, to the shoulder, to the ear to outside of the eyebrow.

TE 8

TE 7

TE 6

TE 5

TE 4

TE 3

TE 2

TE 1

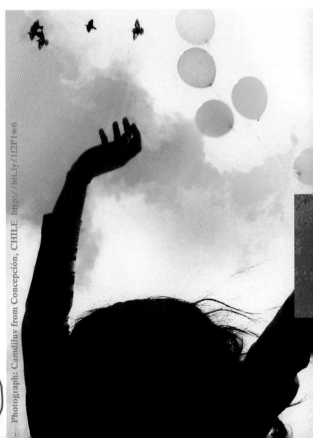

Heart Acu Point

Heart 7-Shen Men-Spirit Gate

Location: On the inner wrist crease, in line with the pinky, on the thumb side of the tendon.

Benefits: Insomnia from over-excitement, anxiety, heart problems or pain, palpitations, mental or emotional imbalances, irritability, or headache.

For acupressure, use your middle or index finger at a 90-degree angle to the points. Apply firm and steady pressure. It may be tender but shouldn't be painful. Hold the point for about 3 minutes. You can also visualize light coming out of your finger and illuminating the meridian and the associated organ.

Small Intestine Acu Point

Small Intestine 3-Hou Xi-Back Ravine

Location: On outside of the hand on the pinky side. When you make a fist, it is the high point on the crease above the pinky.

Benefits: Tinnitus (ringing in the ears), stiff neck, back pain, occipital pain, night sweats, dizziness, earache, sore throat, anxiety, manic depression.

Pericardium Acu Point

Pericardium 6-Nei Guan-Inner Pass

Location: Two thumb widths from the wrist crease on the inner forearm between the two tendons

Benefits: Nausea, motion sickness, hiccups, vomiting, stomach grumbling, abdominal pain or distention. Good for tightness in the chest, palpitations, anxiety, shortness of breath, as well as insomnia

Triple Warmer Acu Point

Triple Warmer 5-Waiguan-Outer Pass

Location: Two thumb widths from wrist crease on midline of outer arm between the two bones

Benefits: Fever, chills, headaches, neck strain, arm, elbow, wrist or finger problems, hand tremors, hearing issues or ringing in the ears.

Time of Day Fire Meridians Peak

Energy travels in the acupuncture organs and meridians throughout the day in a 24-hour period.

Energy peaks in the Heart channel at 11 AM to 1 PM.

I have heard that many heart attacks occur around noon. We are usually digesting lunch at 1–3 pm, so it is important to chew well, as the small intestine has no teeth and can only absorb small molecules of nutrition.

Energy peaks in the small intestine channel at 1 PM to 3 PM.

Energy peaks in the Triple Warmer at 9-11 PM.

Energy peaks in the pericardium channel from 7-9 PM.

Healing Sound for the Heart

Qigong has a healing sound for the major organs. *Ke* is the sound for healing of the heart, and easing heart fire.

STEP 1: Inhale naturally and hold your breath. Raise both arms up from your side, your palms facing down. Relax your shoulders, keeping your wrists and elbows naturally bent and relaxed.

STEP 2: When your arms are even with your shoulders, rotate your palms until they are facing in and circle them towards your chest. Then, rotate your palms until the fingers of both hands are pointing at each other without touching and palms facing down. While holding your breath, imagine leading energy up from your left big toe up the inside of your left leg and into your abdomen. Continue up into you heart.

STEP 3: Exhale and vocalize the sound of *Ke* (*Kurrrr*), (interestingly "coeur" is French for heart) with your mouth half open, tongue touching the bottom of your mouth, and exerting a slight pressure with your jaw. At the same time, lower both palms down to your abdomen. Hold up your anus area and draw your abdomen in. During exhalation, lead energy from your heart down the inside of your left arm to and out at the tip of your little finger. Exhale out all the impurities. Repeat steps 1-3 six times. This completes a set. Do three sets.

Taking Care
of the Heart

＊ Align with your true nature and cultivate your own authenticity.

＊ Have integrity in your relationships, knowing and expressing who you are and what you want.

＊ Spend less time doing things that don't matter to you and with people who don't feed your spirit.

＊ Meditation, prayer, drawing, journal writing, and mindful walking in nature nurtures Shen.

As you balance your heart, your life is infused with a light or glow. You increase illumination, intuition, and insight into your everyday life, guiding your decisions. You will have greater ease in loving, discerning the differences between I and thou, and breaking patterns of codependency.

America
the Toxic

By
Warren King, L.Ac

I had a teenage patient complaining of a tight chest and rapid heartbeat. She noticed it only happened on weekdays, always after a school lunch. She always had what she thought was the healthiest choice, a salad. When she brought her own organic lunch to school, the symptoms disappeared.

Lettuce

Lettuce is one of the top vegetables for high levels of pesticide residues.

Photographs: Department of Agriculture http://bit.ly/1gDYjzN

Cord Blood Study

**In 2004 Environmental Working Group (EWG) tested cord blood of 10 newborns and found an average of 204 chemicals per baby.
A total of 287 different chemicals were found.**

Of the 287 chemicals found:

- 180 cause cancer.

- 217 are toxic to the brain and nervous system.

- 208 cause birth defects or abnormal development in animal studies.

There has been a dramatic rise in autism, Parkinson's and Alzheimer's over the last 20 years, which is likely made worse by toxins.

The EWG only tested for a few hundred out of a possible 90,000 chemicals, so they would have found more if they had tested for them. It cost $10,000 per child to do the testing.

Some of these chemicals, like nonstick chemicals used in clothes, furniture, food wrappers and nonstick pans even showed up in penguins and arctic seagulls.

Toxins bioaccumulate, meaning that those at the top of the food chain get the most concentrated chemicals.

Process of Disease

1. Absorption of toxins

2. Deposition of toxins

3. Degeneration by toxins

The body will try to expel toxins with vomiting, fever, diarrhea, and/or skin rash.

Some toxins are from within the body (like from food allergies, parasites, yeast, poor digestion), and some are from the outside.

In America the Toxic, we are focusing on the external toxins.

Toxins

Toxins block the function of mitochondria, the cells' energy centers. This can cause fatigue. The recent rise of autoimmune diseases reflects the increase of toxicity in the environment.

Most environmental toxins are fat soluble. The liver processes foods and transforms them from being fat soluble to water soluble so they can be eliminated.

Becoming obese may be a sign of toxicity. The body's intelligence may be storing toxins away from major organs because it can't find a way to eliminate them.

Chronic Toxicity Symptoms

- Fatigue
- Sleep disturbance
- Intestinal distress
- Allergies
- Headaches
- Confusion
- Anxiety

Pesticides

5.1 billion pounds of pesticides are used in the
United States every year.

**More than 20,000 pesticides are registered with the
Environmental Protection Agency.**

Pesticides are used on livestock to control insects and are
in their feed as well.

*This is the most common environmental toxin
I see affecting people. You need to get mostly organic,
especially for the dirty dozen. Eating at restaurants
frequently is a real risk.*

The Dirty Dozen

The dirty dozen are the fruits and vegetables with the highest pesticide residues.

1. Apples

2. Strawberries

3. Grapes

4. Celery

5. Peaches

6. Spinach

7. Sweet Bell Peppers

8. Nectarines (Imported)

9. Cucumbers

10. Cherry Tomatoes

11. Snap Peas (Imported)

12. Potatoes

Pesticides and GMOs

The average child in the United States between the ages of 6 and 11 has been found to have 4 times the acceptable levels of pesticides.

Now GMO plants like corn produce a pesticide in every cell of the plant.

This pesticide, or Bt toxin, has been found in 93% of pregnant women and 80% of umbilical blood of babies. This can create learning problems, allergies, digestive problems and auto immune diseases.

I have noticed, as have other healers, that many patients who feel unwell even though they eat a very limited and strict diet, go to Europe and eat a rich, gluten full wide diet and feel great and then feel poorly when back in the US even when eating healthy food.

Genetically Modified (GM) Crops

Some crops are genetically engineered to withstand herbicides such as Roundup®. This has led to an increased use of chemicals and the development of resistant super weeds that nothing can kill.

- 88% of soybeans
- 91% of corn
- 100% canola oil

70% of processed foods contain GM ingredients.

Animals get fatter when fed GM corn...and so do we.

Are organic foods better for you?

Commercial vegetables are larger than they used to be, but **have 5% – 40% fewer minerals, such as magnesium, iron, calcium, and zinc than 50 years ago... and they aren't as tasty.**

Healthier soil leads to higher levels of nutrients in crops.

Children with higher levels of pesticides had higher risk of ADHD.

Organic fruits and vegetables have 40% more antioxidants. Organic milk has 90% more.

USDA ORGANI

Photo: Linsenhejhej http://bit.ly/1fdgewF

Rats and Organics

In 2005 scientists compared the health of rats fed conventional diets to those on organic diets. Rats fed organic foods had:

- Improved immune system status.

- Better sleeping habits.

- Less weight and slimmer appearance.

- Higher vitamin E content in their blood.

Animal Foods

Grazing and growing feed for livestock uses 70% of all agricultural land and 30% of the earth's landed surface.

CAFOs: (Concentrated Animal Feeding Operation)
- Produce enormous amounts of sewage, methane, and other pollutants.

- Can house hundreds to millions of animals.

They are not the image of farms that we grew up with. These are animal concentration camps. Egg-laying machine chickens are stacked in cages, unable to move. Hogs are housed in cages where they can't even turn around, biting at the metal bars as they go insane. Cows are now fed GMO corn and soy instead of grass, which their digestive tracts are not made to digest.

Animal Products

Turkeys are often so cramped that they will peck each other to death, and as a result their beaks can be cut off.

Animals that like to be clean are caked in their own waste.

Many animals are diseased, and have a continuous feeding of antibiotics, hormones, and pesticide-laden grain which all end up in the milk, meat, and eggs.

Hormones are used to make larger animals, or produce more milk.

Animals are often cut open while still alive, and all that pain and suffering is part of the meat you eat.

Bred to Be Huge!

Look at this image showing how we have bred chickens to become gigantic in a much shorter time span. Some cannot even walk. If we eat this kind of food often, it's no surprise that our children become obese at younger and younger ages. The hormones, antibiotics, and arsenic fed to them to make them fat can do the same to us.

Photo: Poultry Science

Farmed Fish

84% of seafood in the United States is imported, and half of that is farm raised.

Every Atlantic salmon must eat 5 times its weight in fish. To save on fish they are now eating barley, corn, and soybeans, not their native diet.

Fish feed contains chemicals and antibiotics as well to deal with health issues from overcrowding and filth.

Common environmental toxins like dioxins and PCBs are 7 times higher in farmed than wild fish, which have high levels of toxicity already.

Salmon are not supposed to be kept in pens like couch potatoes. They are supposed to swim up rivers and waterfalls. Sitting around eating all day to get fat quickly is what they do, and that is what happens to those who eat them.

Now the fish industry wants to genetically engineer salmon with an eel-like fish to produce a creature that is twice as big as a normal salmon and matures in half the time.

Humanely Raised Animals

If you decide to eat animal foods, vote with your pocketbook.

Animals should have space to do what they like to do in nature.

They should eat what they eat in nature. Cows like grass and pasture, not genetically modified corn and soy.

They should be killed by the quickest and most painless methods possible.

Chickens like to peck and scratch the ground and look for insects. Pigs like to root around on the ground, some studies suggest they are smarter than dogs.

I saw one study where a dog and pig were trained to use a computer joystick and when they scored they got food. The pig was able to do it every time after it learned how. The dog had to be retaught every time.

Preservatives

Preservatives keep food from going bad.

There are time-tested methods such as using salt, vinegar, sugar, and ascorbic acid.

But today, **most preservatives are synthetic and toxic and tumor causing.**

They prevent bacterial, mold, and yeast growth, preserve color and flavor, and keep foods fresh by preventing oxidation and rancidity.

Most chemical preservatives affect the nervous system, and some have an impact on reproductive health, or weaken the immune system.

Photo: Hoda Varian https://bit.ly/190ueJ3

Modern Preservatives

Nitrates enhance flavor and preserve color, mostly in meats. **They are carcinogenic and should be avoided, especially for children.**

Sulfites and sulfur dioxide are derived from coal tar. They keep food from browning and are found in dried fruit and wine, and can cause headaches, hyperactivity, and asthma.

BHA and BHT are considered the most dangerous preservatives and are outlawed in many other countries. They are carcinogens and have been found to cause stomach cancer. Baby mice exposed to these preservatives weighed less, slept less, and fought more. Although these preservatives are found in low levels in an individual food, over the years they accumulate and can cause serious problems.

Benzoic acid and sodium benzoate are found in many products and also cause hyperactivity and can cause eye and skin irritation. They are found in acidic foods like dressings, carbonated drinks, pickles, condiments, and jams and jellies.

Artificial Colors

One of the most widely used and dangerous additives

In Europe, warning labels are required on foods with dyes, but not in the United States.

Many dyes cause tumor growth in rodents and some create hyperactivity in children.

Every year, food manufacturers pour 15 million pounds of artificial food dyes into U.S. foods.

I notice that most parents don't think twice about giving their children rainbow-colored cereal or fluorescent-blue drinks and slushies, and they don't consider bright orange cheese puffs out of the ordinary, either. But the same people often make sure their pets are eating all-natural dog food.

Blue #1 causes kidney cancer in mice.

Blue #2 also causes cancer, especially brain tumors in male rats.

Citrus red #2 is found in Florida orange skins and causes bladder cancer in rodents.

Green #2 causes increase in bladder and testes tumors in male rats, but at least your prescription drugs have a nice color!

Red #3, the dye that makes maraschino cherries bright red, has been recognized as a thyroid carcinogen by the FDA since 1990.

Red #40 is the most commonly consumed dye and may accelerate immune system tumors and cause allergies and hyperactivity.

Yellow #5 can cause hyperactivity and other behavioral changes in children.

Yellow #6 causes adrenal tumors and severe reactions in some people.

MSG

Monosodium Glutamate (MSG) is added to food to enhance flavor. It produces many symptoms in sensitive people.

MSG is a form of concentrated salt added to foods to enhance the flavor.

It is particularly harmful to the nerves and brain and may be linked to Alzheimer's and Parkinson's disease.

It's dangerous because it can cause:

- migraine headaches
- balance difficulties
- disabling arthritis
- serious depression
- behavioral problems in children
- severe shortness of breath, asthma attacks, and heart irregularities

MSG is a very toxic substance, particularly to the developing brain, especially in the developing fetus.

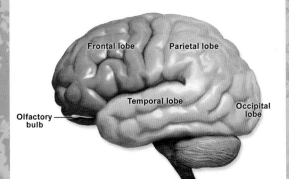

Image: Blausen.com staff, "Blausen gallery 2014". Wikiversity Journal of Medicine. DOI:10.15347/wjm/2014.010. ISSN 20018762

The amount of MSG used in food has doubled every decade since it was first used in the 1940s.

It is hidden in many foods under innocuous-sounding names. The food industry tends to rename MSG to avoid public scrutiny. There are approximately 40 names for it, including the words "hydrolyzed" or "autolyzed" yeast or "yeast extract." It may be derived from a fermented protein like soy protein or whey protein.

Under current FDA regulations, when MSG is added to a food, it must be identified as monosodium glutamate in the label's ingredient list. However, if MSG is part of a spice mix that is purchased by another company, the manufacturer does not have to list the ingredients of that spice mix and may use the words "flavorings" or "spices."

Artificial Sweeteners

Artificial sweeteners are now found in thousands of products and should be avoided.

Being around 200 times sweeter than sugar, artificial sweeteners negatively affect blood sugar and create more sweet cravings. Nobody really loses weight on these products.

These sweeteners trick the body into thinking that carbs are coming, so the pancreas releases insulin, causing a yo-yo effect in the blood sugar.

They also make you used to food being so sweet that you can't taste the subtle sweetness found in vegetables and grains.

Artificial sweeteners have been found to throw off the balance of bacteria in the intestines, leading to diabetes and weight gain, the exact things people who take them are trying to avoid.

NutraSweet®, or **aspartame,** has had the most reported adverse effects, largely on the nervous system. It is transformed into formaldehyde in the body and has been found in the liver, kidneys, and brains of those who consume it. It can also affect vision. It is called an excitotoxin because it stimulates nerve and brain cells to the point that they may die.

AcesulfameK, brand names: Sunett®, Sweet One®, is the least studied and may cause cancer and damage to the organs, so it is best to avoid it.

Sucralose or **Splenda®**, is a denatured sugar that has added chlorine. It has been shown to shrink the thymus, which I find is a key to immunity and fighting cancer. It damages the liver and kidneys and reduces the beneficial bacteria, which is a key to immunity and digestive health.

Saccharine or **Sweet'N Low®** used to have a warning for bladder cancer, which has been removed, but it is really not safe to use.

Fluoride

Fluoride is found in 70% of our water supply.

There is no difference between rates of tooth decay in fluoridated and non-fluoridated water.

The level of fluoride in tap water is 250 times the level found in breast milk.

Fluoride is a by-product of fertilizer manufacturing and is contaminated with lead, arsenic and aluminum.

Fluoride lowers the IQ of children.

Reverse osmosis removes fluoride from the water. Most other filters do not.

Cities are starting to decide to save money and people's health by stopping fluoridation. Some cities have lowered the fluoride level because children were getting permanently mottled teeth.

When I go to the dentist I have them polish my teeth with pumice and I forgo the fluoride treatments.

Tap Water and Chlorine

The chlorine in tap water combines with organic matter in the water and creates chlorine disinfection by-products, which are potent carcinogens.

Chlorine kills bacteria, including beneficial flora in the intestines. It can also cause bone loss, allergies, asthma, birth defects and hardening of the arteries.

Drugs are found in tap water from urine, which doesn't filter them out.

Fish are having their sex changed from birth control pills entering the water. In studies, half of all male fish were making eggs in one river, and 1/4 had damaged sperm. This may be responsible for the rise in human infertility.

Drink and cook only with filtered or spring water.

Photo: Angelsharum http://bit.ly/1fdgewF

Mercury

Dental fillings are often called "silver fillings," but they are more than 50% mercury. The mercury constantly off-gasses and accumulates in the body.

If one filling was dissolved in a 10-acre lake, there would be an advisory not to eat fish from that lake.

Mercury is also found in many fish. This is often caused by waste from the burning of coal for energy, which ends up in lakes and rivers.

The new fluorescent light bulbs contain mercury as well.

The most serious and hard-to-treat diseases are very often from the mercury in dental fillings.

Some very bad cases of eczema and psoriasis have been cured after removing mercury and detoxifying the body.

Mercury should be illegal to use in dentistry.

*I had a patient who thought she had Multiple Sclerosis.
I found that it was actually mercury poisoning from fish.
She had been in Florida and eaten grouper every day. More
mercury bio-accumulates when larger fish eat smaller fish.*

Arsenic

Treated wood used to be a source of arsenic.

Now arsenic is fed to commercial chickens to make them grow bigger and give them a pink color. Arsenic kills parasites so the chickens grow larger. It damages their blood vessels, giving the meat a pinker color.

Levels in chickens are 6–9 times higher than the maximum level allowed in drinking water, and chicken litter is now fed to cows! One farmer in Arkansas spread chicken litter on his land, and arsenic started showing up in the houses nearby.

Now rice is showing up high in arsenic. Some of it is in the soil where they used to grow cotton, which was treated with pesticides that contained arsenic.

Aluminum

Aluminum is toxic to the nervous system. It is found in cookware, aluminum foil, deodorants and antiperspirants, table salt, vaccines, and aluminum cans.

The outer breast near the underarm is where most breast cancers occur, leading some to surmise that antiperspirants may play a role in breast cancer. Aluminum shows up concentrated in the brains of Alzheimer's patients.

I prefer stainless steel, ceramic and enamel-coated cookware.

Personal Care Products

A person is exposed to 126 chemicals a day through personal care products.

Phthalate plasticizers, paraben preservatives, the antibiotic triclosan, synthetic musks, and sunscreen can disrupt hormones.

The Environmental Working Group has a cosmetics database called Skin Deep®, which lets you search over 75,000 ingredients for safety.

NBC TV Producer Did Her Own Experiment

A producer for Dateline NBC took urine tests for herself and her 2 children for BPA, phthalates, and triclosan, "the deadly three." These chemicals have been found in 90% of the population.

Her levels were high on the tests. Her 6-month-old baby had 10 times the average of triclosan (an antibiotic found in antibiotic soaps), and her toddler had 100 times the average. These chemicals are found in hand soaps, canned foods, cash register receipts, paper money, plastic containers, and more. Hormone disrupters like Bisphenol A can cause childhood obesity, ADD, autism and infertility.

Levels of these chemicals went way down when the family ate organic foods and used natural beauty and cleaning products. They skyrocketed again when the producer intentionally went back to her old ways of microwaving, drinking diet soda, and using toxic products to see if the test results would go back up.

Photo: Leslie Seaton   http://bit.ly/190ueJ3

EMFs

EMFs (electromagnetic fields) are a new source of toxicity for many people. Cell phone towers, cell phones, computers, Wi-Fi, Bluetooth, cordless phones, electrical appliances and wiring can interfere with the body's cells, signaling, and communication.

EMFs can lower immunity, melatonin, thyroid and testosterone levels. And they accelerate the growth of mold and viruses.

- A teenager had a cyst on his pituitary gland that was from a wire in his mouth, along with hours a day spent playing video games with a Bluetooth headset.

- A woman who kept her cell phone in her bra developed a breast tumor in the shape of a rectangle.

Every week I have to tell a few people that they are being affected by Wi-Fi and they should at least turn it off while they sleep. I advise people to keep cell phones out of their bedrooms while sleeping. I rewired my whole house to get rid of EMF's.

Cell Phones

In brain scans you can see how radiation enters the brain. Radiation goes especially deep in children. **So minimize the cell phone use with children, and use a landline phone when possible.**

It is best to keep your cell phone off your body when you're not using it, and use it as a speaker phone to keep it away from your brain.

Cell phones have been shown to have a link to DNA damage, along with…

- Memory loss
- Alzheimer's disease
- Cancer
- Breakdown of the brain's defenses
- Reduced sperm count

When reception is bad and you have only a few bars, the phone must send out a stronger signal. **Keep your cell phone away from your body when it's on. It is best to limit cell phone usage to brief messages, texting, and short conversations.**

Microwaves

Plastic containers or tableware can leach into the food. Plastics can mimic estrogen in the body and create health problems.

Microwaves can damage food on a molecular level. Microwaves destroy the energetic level of foods by 60%–90%, and harm the vitamins, minerals, and enzymes in the food.

Some research says there has been more tumor formation especially in the stomach and intestines that may be due to microwave use.

There is a Japanese saying: "Where there is a front, there is a back. The larger the front, the larger the back." This means that things that may seem easy and enjoyable now may lead to larger, more costly problems later.

Macrobiotic educator Michio Kushi used to say: "Give your microwave to your best enemy or the military."

Detoxification

There are many methods of detoxification that can help remove toxins from the body.

The key is to open up the drainage routes that carry waste out of the body. They are called emunctories. The primary emunctories are the kidneys, liver, intestines, and lungs. Secondary elimination occurs through the skin, mucous membranes, nose, genitals, and joints.

Most symptoms that people take pills for are actually the body trying to detoxify. Taking pills may just cause suppression of the symptoms, but suppression works temporarily and the body will find another exit. If all exits are closed, then toxins may end up in areas of less importance like fat cells, joints, gallbladder, uterus or breasts, where the toxins may eventually cause further complications and disease.

163

Tools to Detoxify

Fasting
Cleansing
Drinking clean water
Green, leafy vegetables
Seaweed
Lymphatic massage
Exercise
Colonics
Saunas

Biochemical methods: Herbs, vitamins, minerals.

Energetic methods: Laying on of hands, acupuncture, auricular medicine (ear acupuncture), homeopathy, Qigong.

For 20 years I have been working with over 9,000 people on detoxifying. Some have a stronger detoxifying ability than others, but all can be healthier by avoiding toxins when we have a choice, and consciously working on detoxifying our bodies. You don't have to be a fanatic. Our bodies know how to detoxify, but remember that avoiding toxins is especially important for the fetus and children.

Can Toxins Make You Less Beautiful?

Viktor Yushchenko was poisoned by political enemies in Russia with dioxin, a common environmental toxin.

So if you still don't want to avoid toxins for all the myriad health reasons, or the shortening of your lifespan, then at least do it for vanity's sake!

~ The End ~

organs@warrenking.com
loveyourorgans.com
Visit our website for a symptom questionnaire
for the 5 elements, recipes for each element, and more.

WARREN KING, L.Ac

15612 Highway 7, Suite 252
Minnetonka, MN 55345

(952) 930-3575

www.warrenking.com
organs@warrenking.com
www.facebook.com/warrenkinghealing